EMERGENCY

Ian R

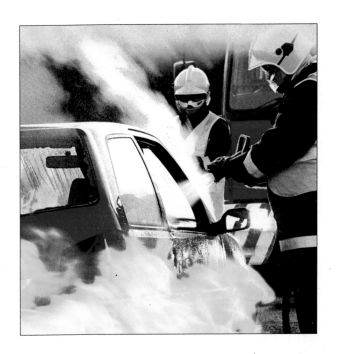

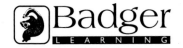
Badger
LEARNING

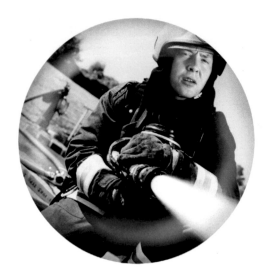

Lexile® measure: 590L
For more information visit: www.Lexile.com

Brainwaves Blue
Emergency
ISBN 978 1 74164 024 3

Copyright © 2005 Blake Publishing
Reprinted 2006, 2010, 2014, 2015
Lexile Copyright © 2013 MetaMetrics, Inc.

Badger Publishing Limited
Oldmedow Road
Hardwick Industrial Estate
King's Lynn PE30 4JJ
Telephone: 01438 791037
Website: www.badgerlearning.co.uk

2 4 6 8 10 9 7 5 3 1

Series publisher: Katy Pike
Series editors: Sophia Oravecz and Garda Turner
Designer: Cliff Watt

Printed by Face Communications (2007) Ltd

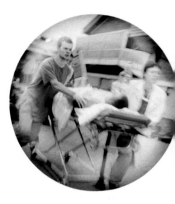

CONTENTS

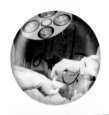

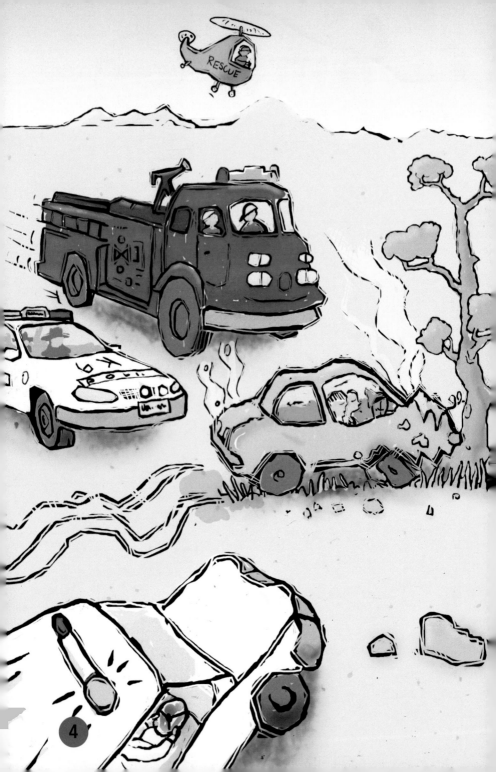

4

Crash!

Brakes squeal. A car swerves.
A surprised kangaroo hops off the
road. But it's too late, the driver
has lost control.

The car skids and hits a tree. It sits
there, crumpled. Steam comes from
the engine. Petrol and oil ooze onto
the ground. Inside, a woman moans.
The man in the driver's seat is quiet
and still.

It is time for the emergency
services to do their jobs.

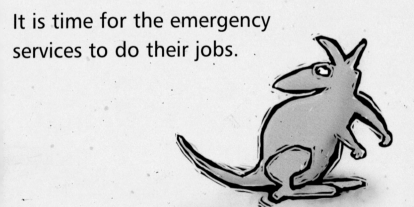

At the Scene

A driver sees the crash and rings for an ambulance. Within 20 minutes it is at the scene. The police and a fire-engine go too. The ambulance workers check each person. They need to know how hurt they are.

One is shaken, has some deep cuts and a broken arm. The other looks bad. He is **unconscious**. The ambulance workers are worried. What if he has internal injuries? He needs a doctor, and fast.

Ambulance workers give injured people strong painkillers at the scene to reduce their discomfort.

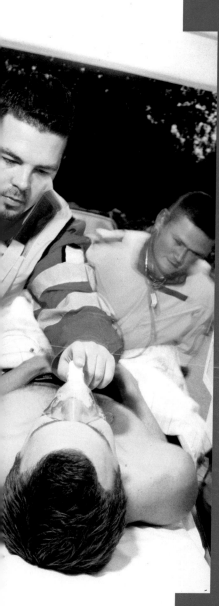

Who does what at a crash site?

Police: Keep onlookers away. Interview witnesses or those involved, if they are not injured, to try to find out what caused the accident. Direct other traffic around the crash site.

Ambulance: Give first aid or emergency treatment to injured people. Inform hospital of injuries to victims. Transport victims to hospital.

Fire brigade: Put out any fires that the accident may have caused. Make sure that any oil or petrol on the road is cleaned up. These can make the road slippery and lead to more accidents.

We Need a Doctor!

The ambulance workers ring the closest hospital. They tell the hospital workers that the man is badly hurt. He needs emergency care before he can be moved. The hospital quickly sends a doctor.

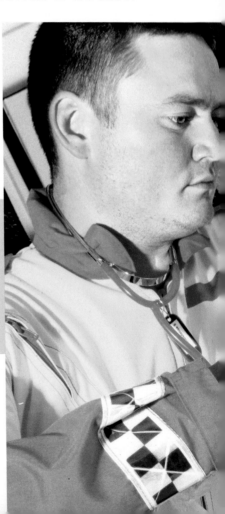

Accident victims are often unconscious and can't breathe properly. Ambulance workers give them oxygen.

Another ambulance worker treats the hurt woman. As well as the broken arm and cuts, she is in **shock**. She is also worried about her friend. He is still unconscious.

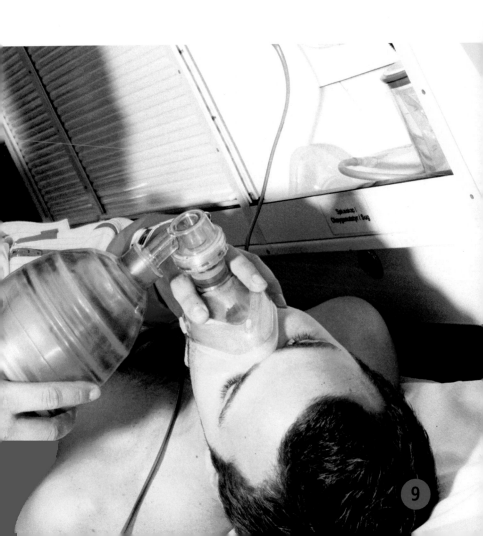

Racing to Hospital

The doctor has arrived and begins working on the man.

Another ambulance arrives. It takes the woman to the hospital's casualty ward.

Back at the scene of the crash, the doctor has finished. He needs more help, and quickly. The ambulance rushes the patient to hospital — lights flashing and siren screaming.

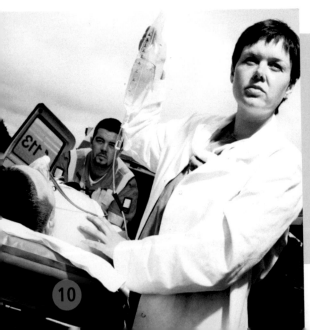

If a doctor is at the scene, they will often travel to the hospital in the ambulance in case the patient's condition suddenly worsens.

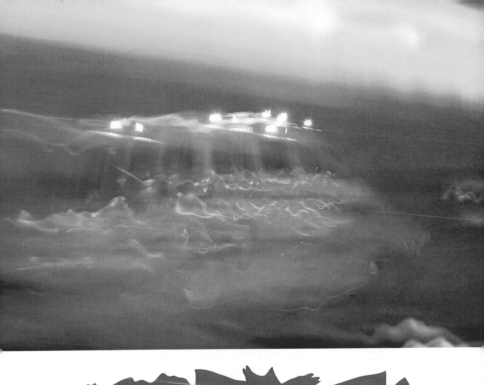

What happens when you call '000'?

1. Person calls '000'.
2. Operator asks if they want Police, Fire or Ambulance.
3. Person put through to service.
4. Operator takes details and sends the appropriate emergency service or services.

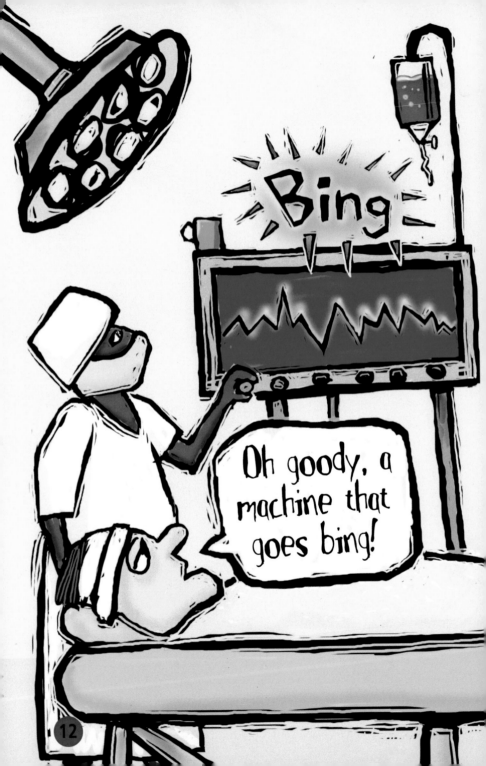

At the Hospital

The siren screams as the ambulance arrives.

The doctors and nurses at the hospital are ready. An operating theatre has been prepared. They know that the man in the ambulance is very badly hurt. It is their job to try to save his life.

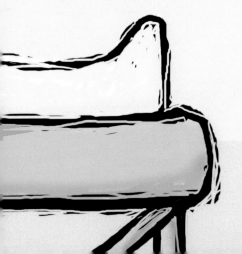
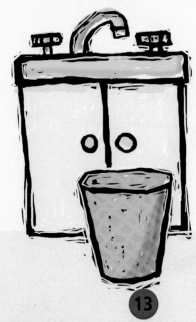

No Time to Lose

The ambulance pulls up. The officers quickly wheel the patient to the theatre. It's a short journey that they've done many times. Their job ends. Now, the hospital medical staff takes over.

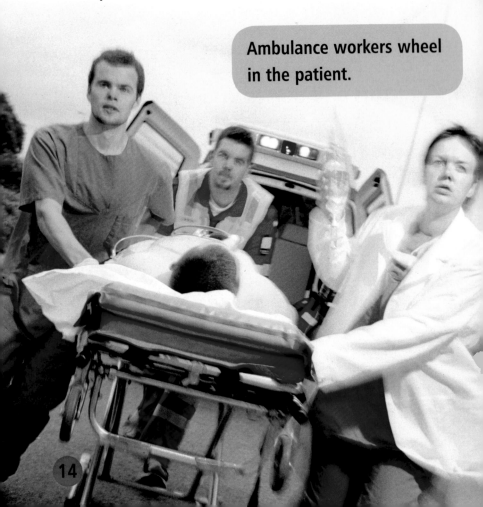

Ambulance workers wheel in the patient.

The patient is soon under an **anaesthetic**. Nurses and the anaesthetist watch the patient's **vital signs**. Surgeons go to work. They need to treat a **ruptured** organ.

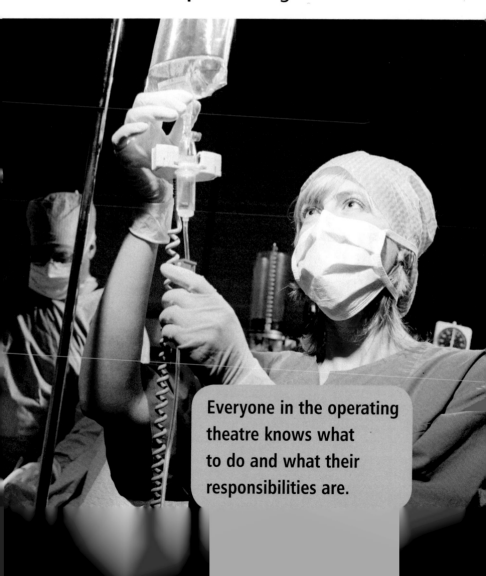

Everyone in the operating theatre knows what to do and what their responsibilities are.

Medical Alert!

A lot can go wrong during an emergency operation. That's why doctors and nurses have some tricks up their sleeves.

If a patient's heart stops, they use machines and drugs to try to get it to beat again. A patient who has lost a lot of blood gets a **transfusion**. Machines can also be used to breathe for patients.

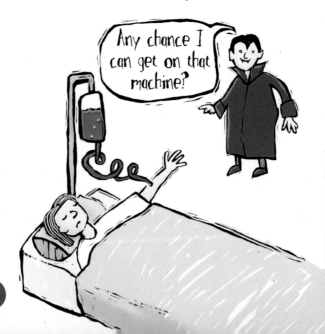

Any chance I can get on that machine?

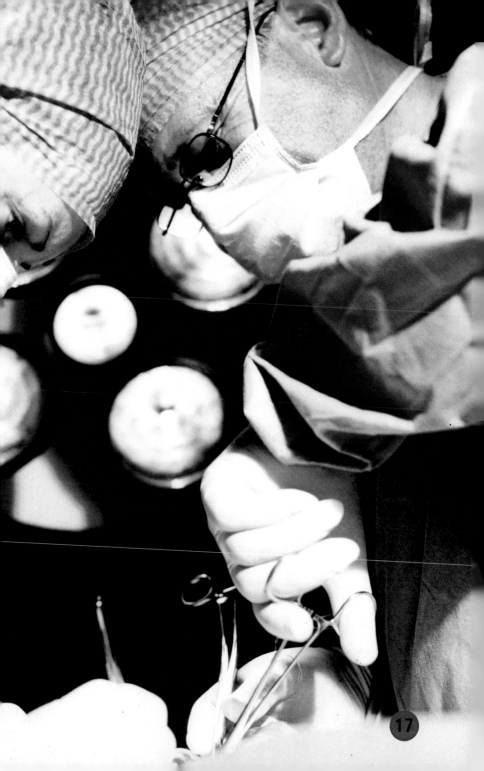

Casualty Care

In the **casualty ward**, nurses take care of the hurt woman. Her arm is **X-rayed**. She is ready for a doctor to stitch her cuts and set the broken bone. If the hospital is very busy she will have to wait. Badly hurt people are looked after first.

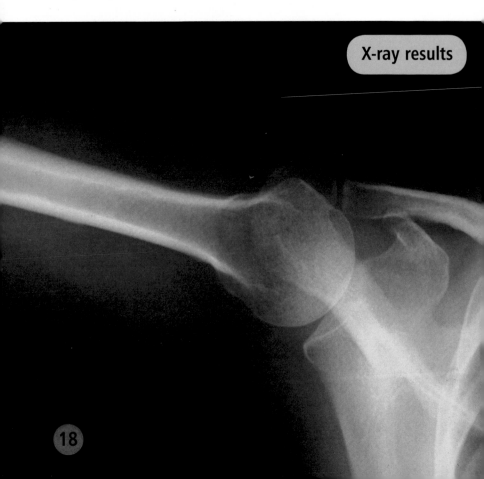

X-ray results

The nurses ask the woman all about her medical history. This will help the doctor work out the best way to treat her.

What is triage?

This is the first step of most visits to a casualty ward. Here someone, usually a nurse, assesses each patient's condition.

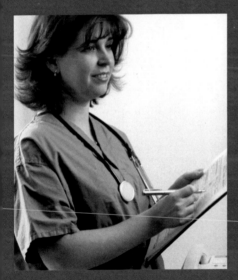

There are three categories: immediately life threatening; urgent but not immediately life threatening; and less urgent. Patients are then seen in that order.

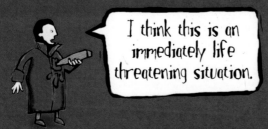

I think this is an immediately life threatening situation.

Quiet Time

Hours after the car hit the tree, the emergency is over. Both of the patients are recovering. However, the man will spend many days in hospital before he can go home.

The police write up their report on the accident. The ambulance workers respond to more calls. The firefighters are back at the station, relaxed but ready. There are no emergencies, for now.

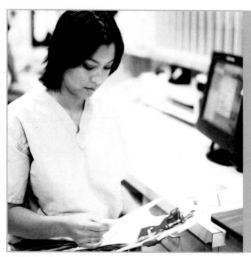

Emergencies aren't all action. All the emergency teams will have to write reports and complete other paperwork about the day's events.

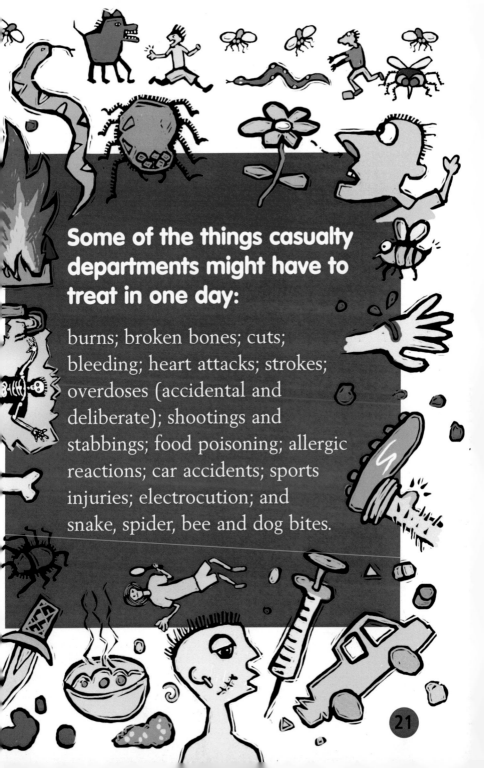

Some of the things casualty departments might have to treat in one day:

burns; broken bones; cuts; bleeding; heart attacks; strokes; overdoses (accidental and deliberate); shootings and stabbings; food poisoning; allergic reactions; car accidents; sports injuries; electrocution; and snake, spider, bee and dog bites.

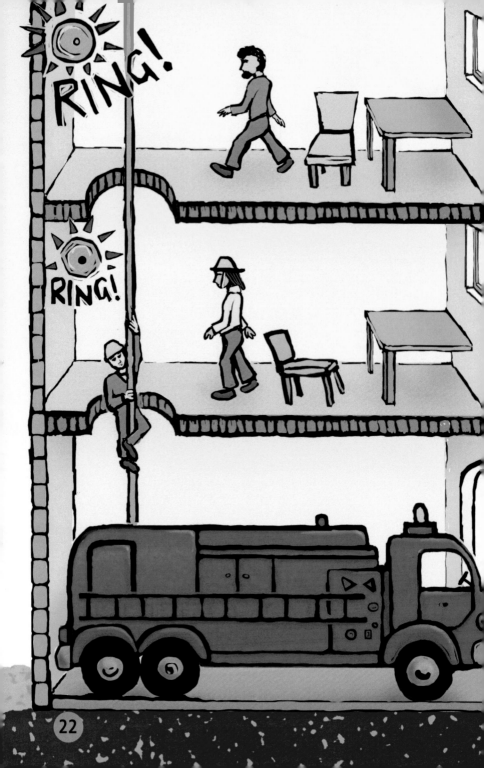

fire! fire!

Bells start ringing. Firefighters rush into action. They slide down poles and put on helmets. They leap into the fire truck, siren screaming, and drive.

It doesn't always happen like that. But a fire is an emergency. Firefighters have to be ready to race to a fire, put it out and save anyone in danger.

The Flame Game

Fires happen almost anywhere. Houses, factories, cars and trucks can all catch fire. In big emergencies, many fire crews are needed to fight the blaze.

Q: What did one flame say to another flame?

A: Let's go out tonight.

Fire crews have two main jobs in an emergency. Firstly, they try to save the lives of anyone in danger. Then, they try to save property and stop the fire from spreading.

Fire crews have sometimes been called to such dangerous jobs as putting out fires in fireworks factories!

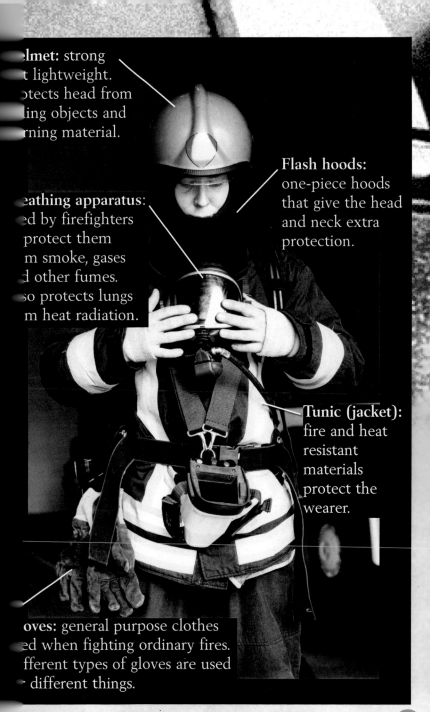

lmet: strong
t lightweight.
otects head from
ing objects and
rning material.

Flash hoods:
one-piece hoods
that give the head
and neck extra
protection.

eathing apparatus:
ed by firefighters
protect them
m smoke, gases
d other fumes.
so protects lungs
m heat radiation.

Tunic (jacket):
fire and heat
resistant
materials
protect the
wearer.

oves: general purpose clothes
ed when fighting ordinary fires.
fferent types of gloves are used
different things.

Blazing Away

When a house is on fire, the crew will first find out if anyone is inside. Once everyone is safe, the fire fight begins. The crew uses special hoses. The flames are hit with thousands of litres of water.

Eventually, the fire is out. Steam rises from the burnt area. The air is smoky, making it hard to breathe. Onlookers cough. They wipe their watering eyes. An ambulance is on the scene. The ambulance workers treat one of the fire crew for **smoke inhalation**. The fire is out, but there is still work to be done.

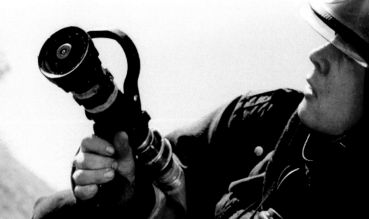

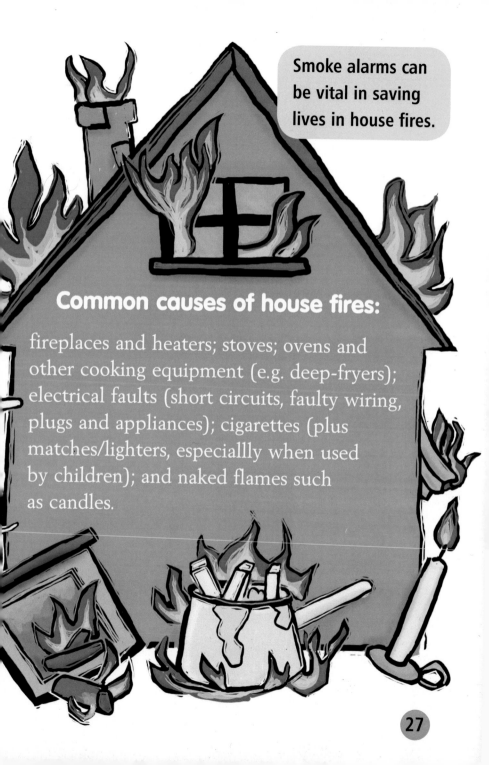

Smoke alarms can be vital in saving lives in house fires.

Common causes of house fires:

fireplaces and heaters; stoves; ovens and other cooking equipment (e.g. deep-fryers); electrical faults (short circuits, faulty wiring, plugs and appliances); cigarettes (plus matches/lighters, especiallly when used by children); and naked flames such as candles.

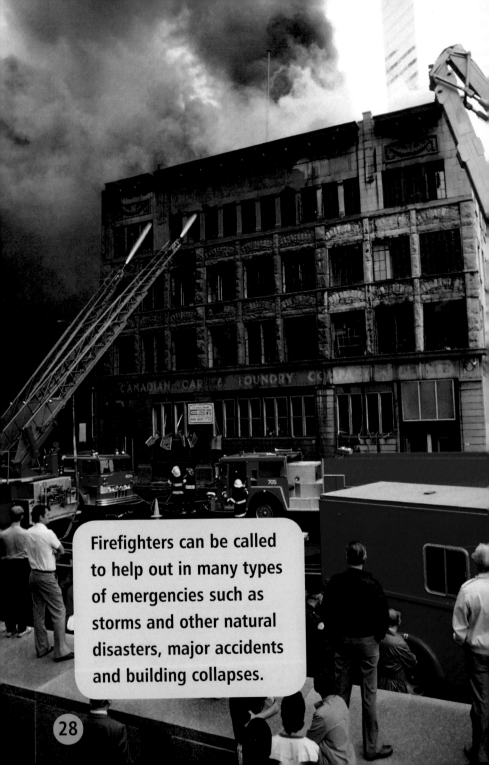

Firefighters can be called to help out in many types of emergencies such as storms and other natural disasters, major accidents and building collapses.

Clean-up Crew

Now that the fire is out, it is time for the clean-up. Firefighters organise for gas and electricity to be cut off. They also try to work out what caused the fire.

Sometimes, they decide that a fire was not an accident. In these cases the police help. They look for clues. They try to find out who started the fire and why. The emergency teams are all busy keeping us safe.

Fire escape plan

A fire escape plan could help save your life or that of others. Schools, workplaces and homes should all have a fire escape plan. A plan includes things such as the different ways out of a space or room, safe meeting places and the location of fire extinguishers.

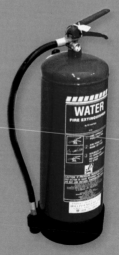

Fact File

The fastest fire engine is the Florida-based Hawaiian Eagle. It's a rocket-powered 1941 truck that has hurtled along at 655 km/h.

Is there a fire on the Moon?

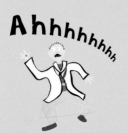

Ahhhhhhhh

Don't work in emergency services if you have haemophobia or nosocomephobia. The first is a fear o blood, the second a fear of hospitals!

Now this is a pile up

Big, car pile-ups can happen when an accident occurs on a busy road. Ninety-eight smashed cars blocked America's Interstate 70 for nearly a kilometre after a major pile-up in 1998. Thirty-seven people were taken to four different hospitals but no-one was killed.

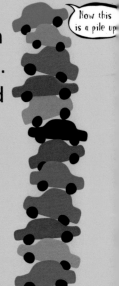

Glossary

anaesthetic	drugs used so people don't feel pain during an operation
casualty ward	hospital area where emergency cases are looked after
ruptured	broken or burst
shock	when your body isn't working properly because of injuries
smoke inhalation	to breathe in smoke
transfusion	giving a person extra blood
unconscious	not aware of what is happening around you
vital signs	heart beat, blood pressure and other signs that show someone's health
x-rayed	having a picture taken of inside the body

Index